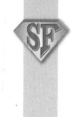

MW01253936

Contents

Are you ready to supercharge your diet?
Ready to cast aside the foods that are not doing your body
and brain any favors?
Ready to choose widely from this list
of the top 50 superfoods and ramp up the nutrition
in your food and drink choices?

It's easy!

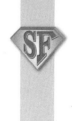

Introduction

So What Is a Superfood?

Some foods are simply more nutritious, better for you, *more packed with the good stuff*. These are the superfoods. And if we all ate more of those foods, we'd be healthier, happier, and, very probably, wealthier and wiser, too.

Healthier because our bodies absolutely need protein, minerals, vitamins, good carbohydrates and fats, antioxidants, and much, much more to function optimally.

Happier because the brain needs all that good stuff too, especially the good fats and vitamins.

Wealthier because we won't be spending heaps of money on either:

- bulk junk food that leaves you literally starving for vitamins and minerals, locked into a cycle of overeating to try to give your body what it craves and needs, or

- bottles of expensive supplements; it's well known that generally our bodies absorb far more nutrients from real, whole foods than from anything in a capsule.

Wiser because of that better-functioning brain and because we know for sure that overprocessed foods and junk foods dull the mind as well as the body!

It's about Quality *and* Quantity

It's all very well knowing that cloves have the highest amount of excellent polyphenolic antioxidants, and by a huge margin. But unless you are going to eat 100 g at a time, are they really that useful? Have you ever tried to eat 100 g of cloves?!

It's better to know that drinking four to five cups of tea a day is also going to deliver a great antioxidant boost. Or perhaps to know that a daily diet featuring an *abundance of the fruit and vegetables* listed in this book will give you *so* much more nutrition than the *occasional expensive handful* of the next trendy so-called superfood to come along.

It's also important to understand that some fruits and vegetables are better than others, as are some meats, some nuts, and even some drinks and sweet treats.

Isn't Superfood a Term Just Used and Abused by Marketers?

Well, the term does get a bit abused these days. If you see the word "superfood" used in the same sentence as "multi-level marketing," it's probably a good idea to run away screaming.

But seriously, in every food group there are simply some foods that are *so* much more nutritious, *so* much better for you. Very often these have been used as both powerful foods and as medicines for thousands of years. Modern medical research has at last been catching up with the wisdom of the ages to explain why these foods really are superfoods.

For example, when you think of fruits, which ones stand out as the best for you? Believe me, it's not an apple a day that will keep the doctor away.

Think blueberries and raspberries or the mighty black-currant or elderberry instead. And don't just sprinkle them on your porridge! Get into the habit of eating 100 g a day, or even more. That's the way to really pump up your diet. Find the good stuff in every food group and set it squarely in the middle of your plate, bowl, or cup.

Superfoods for Weight Loss

There's a move afoot to concentrate less on what foods we shouldn't eat, and instead to focus on foods we can happily eat more of. Good plan! Eating nutrient-rich foods fills the body up, lets the body know there is plenty of what it needs, and helps stop cravings for unhealthy junk.

Too many people are overweight yet undernourished. There are serious concerns in the medical community about the levels of fiber; vitamins D, A, C, and E; and calcium and potassium in the average diet.

Eat nutrient-rich foods and you won't have to worry about being undernourished. Eat whole nutrient-rich foods and you'll find that they can give you everything your body and brain require and for *far fewer calories* than nutrient-poor foods.

Don't just count calories; make your calories count more!

P.S. Don't forget to move that body too: wiggle, jiggle, dance, hop, skip, jump, or jog. Your heart deserves it, and your brain will thank you, too!

Variety Is the Spice of Life

Don't forget that it's vital to *eat a wide variety of superfoods as well as a wide variety of foods in general.* That's why I've included information on more foods than just the top 50. Read through "The Best of the Rest" section starting on page 57 and eat plenty of those foods, too.

Your body and brain will benefit from *diversity,* from indulging in the thousands of nutrients that foods contain. So consume lots and lots of different fruits, vegetables, nuts, meat, fish, lentils, beans, spices, herbs, and beverages.

Different foods contain different amounts of vitamins and minerals as well as the thousands of phytochemicals and antioxidants that we know are vital for optimum health. It's a simple equation: Eating a wide variety of foods will give you a wide variety of nutrients. Your body needs them!

Your body deserves the best and so does your brain.

So let's celebrate the food that is really good for us.

And let's eat plenty of it!

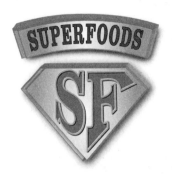

THE
TOP 50
SUPERFOODS

Açaí, Goji, and Inca Berries

This trio of superberries have become in many ways the poster children for superfoods. There's no doubt that all of them are rich in some great nutrients, and they offer excellent antioxidant levels and other health benefits, too. However, they cost a lot more than other fruits and berries. You can get more nutrient bang for your buck by eating larger quantities of other, much-cheaper, berries, fruits, and veggies. But if you're looking for some new tastes, then why not try these berries. They are delicious as well as nutritious.

- Inca berries are a really terrific source of fiber. They are 19 percent fiber by weight, and that's mostly insoluble fiber, which is considered healthy for the gut because they add bulk to the diet, which has a laxative effect and prevents constipation.

- Goji is a good protein source with 12 percent protein (compared with 20 percent protein found in beef).

- All of these berries are a terrific source of antioxidants.

- All of these berries are high in vitamin C.

- All three have high levels of some trace minerals, particularly inca berries, which are high in potassium and phosphorus.

Sprinkle dried berries on top of cereal, or soak them and then add them to breakfast smoothies.

Add to mixed nuts for a terrific between-meal snack.

Use in savory dishes such as stews.

Almonds

Yes, all nuts have a high percentage of fat, but rest assured that most of the fat in nuts is good for you. Indeed, the almond, that old faithful, has some of the highest levels of good fats of all of the nutritious nuts. Almonds are also densely packed with a fantastic variety of vitamins, minerals, protein, and antioxidants, and they've even been proven to work well as part of a weight-loss program. Go nuts!

Almonds are:

- very high in monounsaturated fats
- full of fiber
- high in protein
- high in vitamins E and B-2, as well as the minerals magnesium, potassium, iron, and phosphorous
- a good source of calcium

Also:

- 30 mg of almonds daily has been shown to lower LDL cholesterol.
- Almonds help you feel fuller for longer, so they are a good snack food.
- Nut consumers seem to excrete more fat than people who don't eat nuts.

Buy almonds as fresh as possible, and get into the habit of buying whole almonds with their skins on, for the fiber and extra antioxidants.

Store in airtight containers, ideally in the fridge.

Eat the skin, too.

Toast them yourself; it only takes a few minutes in a hot oven, but the taste is sensational!

Artichoke

Thistles aren't only eaten by donkeys, you know. The artichoke is in fact a thistle and has been a favorite in Mediterranean cuisine for many thousands of years. No, you don't eat the spikes! Nor do you eat the flowers. Rather, you eat the very large edible bud below the flowers. Famed as a medicinal plant, the artichoke is now known to stimulate liver function and to contain compounds that can lower blood cholesterol.

Artichoke is:

- very high in antioxidants
- high in fiber—among the highest of any vegetable
- high in cynarin, which increases the flow of bile, thus aiding digestion
- high in copper
- high in folate and vitamins K and C
- a good source of magnesium, potassium, and manganese

Buy fresh if you can. Choose artichokes that feel heavy and have tightly packed leaves.

Boil or steam the artichokes, then eat them with your fingers.

Peel off the outer leaves and nibble the fleshy edible bottom portion, dipped into butter or hollandaise sauce.

Then remove the fuzzy "choke" and enjoy the succulent and delicately flavored heart.

Mash artichokes with potatoes. Use the mixture to top pizzas or add to warm or cold salads.

Asparagus

This slender stem has been used as both a food and a medicine since the time of the ancient Egyptians. The Romans would eat it fresh in spring then dried throughout the winter. Don't let the very delicate flavor and color of asparagus fool you; it's bursting with vitamins and minerals and deserves a place in every healthy kitchen. Usually seen in its green variety, you might also find white and even purple asparagus these days.

Asparagus is:
- very high in vitamin K
- very high in folate and other B vitamins
- high in vitamins C and E
- high in the amino acid asparagine, named after the asparagus
- high in fiber
- high in a wide variety of antioxidants
- a good source of zinc, iron, manganese, and magnesium
- very low in calories

Buy as fresh as possible; the stalks should snap crisply and be moist and juicy.

Store in the fridge, upright in a jug of water like flowers or wrapped in a damp cloth and placed in a plastic bag.

Eat asparagus raw in salads.

Cook it very quickly; it only needs a very light steam, fry, blanch, or braise.

Try asparagus soup, risotto, and in pastas and frittatas.

Use asparagus as a hangover cure; research suggests it may help break down alcohol in the bloodstream.

Avocado

This fantastic fruit is nutrient dense and filled with the good fats that our bodies and brains need. The luscious avocado is a food that will fill you up and help you feel great. Eating avocado in a colorful salad seems to increase the absorption of all the antioxidants in the other vegetables, probably due to the avocado's good fats.

Avocado is:

- high in vitamins C, K, and E
- rich in folate
- high in fiber—half an avocado contains around 5 g
- high in the carotenoid lutein, great for the skin and eyes

Buy avocados that are blemish free, and don't worry if they are unripe. Avocados never ripen on the tree, they only start to ripen once they are picked.

Ripen your avocados at home—you can pop them in a paper bag with a banana or apple to speed up the process.

Swap butter for avocado on your breakfast toast or lunchtime sandwiches.

Make green smoothies with avocado, banana, mango, milk, spinach, and yogurt. Try it, you'll like it!

Blend avocado and chocolate to make nutritious and delicious desserts. You'll find great recipes online.

Babies tend to love avocado. Give them a great start in life by including it among their first foods.

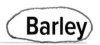

This whole grain is good for so much more than just making beer. Barley is a splendid food that is regaining popularity after being overshadowed by wheat and oats for far too long. Barley can be bought simply hulled, also known as scotch or pot barley, or barley groats, and this is the most nutritious type. It is also commonly sold as pearl barley, meaning the barley has been hulled and then steamed and polished. Although some of the bran has been removed, pearl barley is still a terrific and nutritious grain.

Barley is:

- very high in fiber, which can help reduce blood cholesterol levels as well as being good for the gut flora
- very high in selenium
- high in copper, manganese, and phosphorus
- high in the essential B vitamins

Enjoy boiled or steamed barley in place of rice, potatoes, or couscous. Use three parts water to one part barley and simmer. The slightly nutty flavor and pleasant chewy texture might surprise you.

Make barley risottos, a welcome change from the usual rice.

Add to soups and stews to boost fiber and add nutrients, flavor, and texture.

Substitute barley flour for 25 percent of the wheat flour in cakes, biscuits, and breads.

Beans and Lentils

Raise a cheer for the loveliness of legumes. Loved for their taste and texture, for their versatility, and for their very solid nutritional credentials, beans and lentils are a must-cook for both vegetarians and omnivores.

Beans and lentils are:

- a very low-GI source of carbohydrate
- a useful source of protein that is very easily digested
- a terrific source of soluble fiber, plus amylose, a prebiotic-resistant starch that is good for the gut
- a good source of iron, magnesium, phosphorus, and zinc
- rich in antioxidants

Buy them in cans for simplicity.

Or buy beans dry and then soak and boil them for a much cheaper if more a labor-intensive alternative.

Rinse off the liquid to reduce the salt content of canned beans and lentils.

Replace potatoes and rice with beans or lentils, which are equally filling but much more nutritious.

Vegetarians love beans and lentils and quickly become expert at cooking them.

Don't miss out if you're an omnivore. Add beans or lentils to your stews, soups, or sauces, and enjoy the taste and extra phytochemicals.

Blueberries

Small and round, sweet and tasty, the diminutive blueberry punches well above its weight nutritionally. Just 100 g of the minifruit contains as many antioxidants as two and a half cups of spinach! Buying blueberries doesn't have to break the bank, either. Frozen blueberries are always in season and not too costly given the nutritional benefits.

Blueberries are:

- rated number one of all fruits and vegetables for antioxidant activity
- able to improve memory and motor skills among the aging
- high in vitamin C, B vitamins, beta-carotene, and vitamin E
- high in fiber, very low in sugars
- high in the antioxidant anthocyanins, which can improve heart and circulatory health and eyesight, and can help the body attack urinary tract infections
- a source of resveratrol, which protects the heart, and pterostilbene, which has anticancer effects

Buy fresh or frozen.

Store in the fridge in a container. Do not wash before storing—they can last up to two weeks.

Drink as part of a brain- and body-boosting smoothie.

Eat by the handful; with yogurt, cream, or ice cream; in fruit salads; with cereal; or in muffins.

Add to salads. Yes, try it!

For kids they are an excellent easy and not-too-messy snack.

Broccoli

Broccoli is the groovy green nutritional giant of the cabbage family, much more nutrient-packed than it's leafier cousins. The broccoli we eat is actually a large flower head. Flower power! Broccoli is chock full of antioxidants, several of which are known anticancer agents. Almost all of them have excruciatingly long and complicated names. Broccoli also has anti-inflammatory properties and aids the body's detoxification system. Now there's a new broccoli kid on the block, broccolini, a hybrid of broccoli and Chinese kale with long thin stalks and smaller heads but a similar nutrient profile.

Broccoli is:

- high in vitamin C (one serving gives twice your daily requirement!)
- high in vitamin K, beta-carotene, and B vitamins
- high in folate
- high in fiber, yet very low in calories

Kids often love broccoli. Chop it into little trees and make a forest of broccoli for them.

Eat raw. Yes, it's great raw in salads or to dip into healthy dips—and eaten raw it loses none of its cancer-fighting abilities.

Store in a sealed bag or container in the fridge.

Eat the stalk. Put it in soups or steam, bake, or boil with the heads.

Grows easily in cool climates.

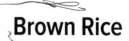

Brown Rice

Is brown rice really a superfood? Well yes and no, to be honest. There are certainly other grains that might seem better at first glance. For example, bulgur wheat hasn't made the Top 50, yet it has a lower GI than brown rice. The tipping point is that brown rice is cheap and universally available, and it has some terrific nutrients. But, crucially, the message is, when you eat rice, eat brown not white. It's so, so much better for you. Opt for lower-GI brown rice, and to reduce the overall GI load, don't eat in huge portions.

Brown rice is:
- super high in manganese
- high in magnesium, phosphorus, and selenium
- high in B vitamins
- a source of fiber

Choose long-grain brown rice as it has a much lower GI than short-grain.

Store in an airtight container in a cool, dry place.

Steaming rather than boiling reduces the GI of rice.

Use one part brown rice to two parts water.

Start your children off on brown rice and they'll love it for life.

Mix lentils into brown rice to make salads and hot dishes.

Serve chicken and fish on a bed of brown rice: It's quick, simple, and totally delicious.

Cabbage

Nobody said you had to look sexy to be a superfood. That's lucky for the humble cabbage, which turns out to be not so humble when it comes to delivering vitamins and minerals, all packaged up with a terrific dose of antioxidants. Learn to unwrap the outer leaves of the more colorful members of the cabbage family and you'll find a storehouse of cancer-fighting nutrients within. Your typical pale green cabbage doesn't pack the punch that the red and deep green varieties do, but it's still a useful vegetable.

Cabbage is:

- very high in vitamin C (it contains even more than an orange!)
- very high in vitamin K
- a useful source of B vitamins
- a useful source of potassium, manganese, iron, and magnesium
- very low in calories

Buy cabbages whole as they start to lose vitamin C as soon as they are cut.

Store in a plastic bag in the fridge.

Choose dark green savoy cabbages or bright red cabbages.

Don't boil the poor old cabbage to death—learn to cook cabbage well: Steam it, braise it, or lightly stir-fry it, and also enjoy cabbage raw.

Kids enjoy biting into chunks of fresh cabbage, munching them like an apple.

Chia

Relatively new on the superfoods market and rather over-hyped by some, chia is nonetheless a terrific addition to a healthy diet. Chia is a seed, but it is often described as a whole-grain food because it contains all the parts of other grains: the bran, the germ, and the endosperm. Generally sold whole, you can also find chia flour. The white and black varieties have a similar nutritional profile.

Chia is:

- very high in healthy omega-3 fatty acids
- low in carbohydrates
- very high in fiber (37 percent of chia is fiber, so it's an easy way to boost your intake)
- high in protein, and it is a complete protein, meaning chia contains all eight essential amino acids—unusual for a plant food
- high in calcium
- a low-GI food
- very filling, so it is excellent for those watching their portions and weight

Buy as seeds, ground seeds, or just the bran.

Eat dry, sprinkled over breakfast cereal.

Eat wet mixed with water to form a gel—mix it into your berry smoothies.

Add chia to many, many dishes to boost their omega-3 levels: salads, burgers, pancakes, muesli bars, stews, and soups.

Mix chia seeds with water to form a gel and use it to replace eggs or oil in baking. Replace some of your white flour with white chia seeds.

Chicken and Turkey

Don't take it for granted: The much-loved chicken really is a superfood. It is a fantastic source of protein, essential to almost every cell in the body. Chicken is low in fat too—not that we don't need fat, but we don't need too, too much of it.

Chicken and turkey are:

- very high in protein (skinless chicken breast is one of the best sources of lean protein in the world)
- high in selenium and phosphorus
- good sources of vitamin B-6, niacin, vitamin A, and vitamin B-12
- the least impactful on the environment of all land-based animal protein foods
- good sources of magnesium
- high in the amino acid tryptophan, which helps regulate the appetite and improves sleep and mood

Buy organic or free-range chicken if you can afford it. The nutritional profile is similar to that of commercially produced chicken but the taste is better (and the chickens are happier and are not routinely fed antibiotics).

Store plenty of chicken in the freezer, then you always have on hand the basics of a healthy meal.

Before cooking, remove the skin—for most dishes you don't need it, and it is very fatty.

Cook thoroughly—poultry cooks very quickly.

Keep your own chickens, as they are not difficult to raise, and they provide eggs.

Drop those apples right now and pick up some citrus fruits instead. Citrus is many times more powerful nutritionally and not just for its very high vitamin C levels. Grapefruits, *Pink* oranges, lemons, limes, satsumas, mandarins, tangerines, and tangelos: eat whichever you like, or better still eat a good variety of all citrus fruits and you'll get a zing from the taste and the nutrients.

Citrus fruits are:

- very low-GI foods
- high in soluble and insoluble fiber, especially the pith
- exceptionally high in vitamin C
- high in folate
- sources of powerful antioxidants (in both the fruit and the skin), some of which are proven anticancer compounds

Buy by the boxful when in season; citrus can be a very cheap purchase.

Don't think that drinking orange juice is doing you as much good as eating the whole fruit. It isn't! Find a blender and liquefy peeled whole fruit with water to make a much better orange juice.

Zest the skin of citrus fruits and use it in yogurt, puddings, cakes, and cookies.

Pink grapefruit is especially antioxidant packed. Its carotenoids impart the pink color, and it has lycopene too.

Add citrus segments to salads. The flavor works well with greens like baby spinach, and the vitamin C helps you absorb the iron.

Kids love a quartered orange in their lunch boxes.

Cocoa and Dark Chocolate

The botanical name of cocoa is *Theobroma cacao,* meaning "food of the gods." The cocoa bean is not actually a bean; it's a nut and like all nuts must be enjoyed in moderation. Pure cocoa powder is of course the best: There's no sugar and no fat, and you can use it in so many ways. But dark chocolate is also pretty good for you, in small quantities. Shhhh…don't tell…there are other foods which are more nutrient dense. Perhaps they should edge dark chocolate out of the Top 50, but we know we love chocolate, and indulging can be good for us in moderation. So if you won't tell, I won't either!

Chocolate is:

- rich in antioxidants called polyphenols, which keep your blood flowing well, can decrease inflammation, and fight cancer
- a source of B vitamins, potassium, and calcium
- very energy dense, especially sweetened chocolate

Buy chocolate in small portions and share with the family.

Eat the very best chocolate and enjoy it enormously—in moderation.

Try whisking cocoa into low-fat milk and warming it for a lovely bedtime drink.

Mix a large spoonful of cocoa powder into a berry smoothie for an extra antioxidant hit.

Add cocoa and protein powder to your hot breakfast cereal for a sensational start to the day.

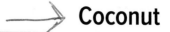

Coconut

Young, mature, green, white, brown and hairy; as flesh, water, milk, or cream: The coconut comes to us in many variations and each has its own nutritional strengths. The coconut is a bit of an overlooked food source, but it's well worth incorporating into more meals and snacks. Coconut is undoubtedly high in saturated fat, and thus needs to be eaten in moderation. However, most of the fats in coconuts are medium-chained saturated fats, which do not raise blood cholesterol levels.

Coconut is:

- super high in fiber
- very high in manganese
- very high in lauric acid, which is a killer of viruses, bacteria, and fungi and which boosts the immune system
- high in selenium, copper, and iron
- energy dense, a good source of calories for those who need to eat plenty of them

Buy fresh young coconuts and use the gel-like flesh for desserts and drinks.

Use lots of coconut in your cakes and cookies and for making fruit and nut truffles and chocolates.

Coconut works well in many soups. Try with beans, pumpkin, chicken, or crab.

Curries really benefit from adding coconut milk or cream. Delicious!

Coffee

Yes, coffee! Drunk in moderation, coffee has many health-boosting properties. Just hold back on sugar and too much milk and you'll be drinking a steaming cup of tasty anti-aging and antidiabetes substances. Yet remember, this superfood comes with a health warning. It can have bad health effects if overconsumed. Stick to three cups of coffee a day and don't drown it in milk or stifle it with sugar. Green coffee is heavily promoted as a weight-loss tool, but there is little credible evidence for this so far.

Coffee is:

- super high in the class of antioxidants called polyphenols. In fact it is the sixth highest per serving after several berries and artichokes
- high in caffeine, which has a stimulating effect on the brain and boosts the metabolism
- a way to significantly reduce the risk of Parkinson's disease in men. It also reduces the risk of Alzheimer's disease and dementia in both men and women
- protective against diabetes
- possibly protective against asthma; however, for those with asthma it has only a very small treatment effect

Buy ground coffee or roasted coffee beans, or buy raw green beans and roast your own.

Don't store coffee in the fridge; it's too moist.

Do store coffee in airtight containers in cool, dry, dark conditions.

Dark Green, Leafy Vegetables

Go green, go as dark green as you can, and enjoy feeling like a nutritional saint. Why is the old advice to "eat your greens" still proving so true in the modern world? It's the phytochemicals. "Phyto" means plant in Greek, so the term just means chemicals found in plants, but the thing is, the deeper a plant's color the more phytochemicals it has. And we're probably only scratching the surface in understanding just how good for us these plant chemicals are.

Swiss chard, kale, watercress, arugula, endive, spinach, beet leaves, and Asian greens like bok choy are just chock full of nutrients. And the great thing is, it isn't difficult to incorporate a lot of these leaves into your daily diet. Just say "salad"!

Leafy greens are:

- high in folate, which is a cancer-fighter and all-around good guy
- low in fat and calories
- very high in vitamin K
- high in iron and calcium (that found in Asian greens is particularly well absorbed)
- high in the carotenoid antioxidants, which are so vital for eye health
- high in beta-carotene, which converts to vitamin A

Buy a lot of leafy greens and add them to everything: salads, stews, and casseroles.

Eat as much as you can. A huge bowl of leaves has so few calories and such great health benefits, fill yourself up and knock yourself out!

Drizzle your salads with a good-quality oil-based salad dressing, as oil will help your body absorb the nutrients.

Do eat leafy greens in preference to taking vitamin A in tablet form. Natural is best.

Learn to love green smoothies, your body will love you for it.

Eggs

The egg is the pocket rocket of the food world. Eggs are low in calories but absolutely packed with essential nutrients. Eggs are quick and easy to cook and can be used in a huge variety of dishes eaten at any time of the day. Eggs are a cheap source of protein, and there's no need to worry too much about the cholesterol. Eat eggs daily and enjoy them.

Eggs are:

- very high in protein—egg protein is of particularly high quality and is very easily digested
- high in vitamin D, providing 20 percent of the recommended daily amount (RDA)
- high in vitamin B-12, selenium, and choline, plus antioxidants, too

Buy organic or free-range if you can. Hens raised outdoors who graze on plants have higher omega-3 fats in their eggs.

Look for omega-3 eggs from hens fed a diet high in omega-3 fats.

Store eggs in their cartons in the coolest part of the fridge, but take them out and use them at room temperature for soft boiling and baking.

For breakfast, eggs have no peer. Fry, scramble, poach, boil, or make French toast.

Excellent as part of any weight-loss strategy.

Flaxseed

Also known as linseed, this deceptively demure and diminutive brown seed hides its light under a bushel. It's the richest plant source of alpha-linolenic acid, from which our bodies make omega-3 oils. You need to know about this little seed, especially if you are a vegetarian. The terrific thing is that we only need a small amount every day to really boost our intake of good fats.

Flaxseed is:

- very high in alpha-linolenic acid
- high in lignans, which lower female estrogen levels, easing symptoms of menopause
- very high in thiamine
- a source of protein

Buy whole seeds or ground seeds, or even ground LSA, which is a mixture of linseed, sunflower seeds, and almonds.

Grind your own flaxseed as you need it, which is easily done in a blender or coffee grinder.

Toast whole or ground flaxseed—imparts a lovely nutty flavor.

Mix ground flaxseed into yogurt and add some berries.

Drink ground flaxseed in your nutrition-packed morning fruit smoothie.

Add to savory dishes like stews, meatballs, and casseroles.

Don't forget to drink lots of water when you eat flaxseed, as it is high in soluble fiber and will absorb water in the digestive tract.

Freekeh

Freekeh, or farik, is a welcome addition to the "new" ancient superfood grains. Freekeh, or roasted young green wheat, was eaten for many thousands of years and then fell out of favor. The younger wheat grain has more protein, vitamins, and minerals than the more mature grain. Freekeh has a delicious nutty flavor; it might almost be described as smoky. Freekeh is sold as a whole grain, a cracked grain, and as freekeh flour. Try it!

Freekeh is:

- higher in protein than the other grains
- high in fiber, containing four times as much as brown rice, most of it insoluble
- a low-GI food
- rich in calcium, iron, potassium, and zinc
- rich in the antioxidants lutein and zeaxanthin, which are important for eye health
- a good source of B vitamins, and vitamins E and C

Use freekeh in place of rice, pasta, and potatoes as a side dish—boil or steam with four to five parts water.

Add freekeh to burgers and soups, or eat as a breakfast cereal.

Use in salads and to make pilafs.

Replace a portion of normal wheat flour with freekeh flour for a nutrient boost in your breads, cakes, and cookies.

Garlic

Garlic has been used as medicine for millennia and it would be silly to stop now. In fact, scientists are now finding and testing the compounds that are so active and healthful. Garlic, in fairly large quantities, for example two to four cloves a day, has been shown to lower "bad" cholesterol and high blood pressure. It is also a proven antibacterial, antifungal, and antiviral agent. Use it lavishly!

Garlic is:

- high in allicin, a sulphur compound that is known to lower cholesterol and prevent tumor growth in the gut
- even thought to boost the sex drive (again, because of the allicin)

Store garlic in a dry, dark place at room temperature, with good air circulation. Do not refrigerate unless you have minced the garlic and put it in an airtight container.

Peel just before using as garlic's potency is reduced when it is exposed to sunlight.

Eat raw, in salad dressing, in dips, or rubbed on toast. Many people simply cut a couple of cloves into pieces and swallow them with a glass of water. Medicinal!

Roast whole bulbs of garlic, then squeeze out the individual cloves and use them in dips, sauces, and salad dressings, or simply spread on toast.

Guava

Guavas are the top of the crop as far as vitamin C is concerned. We need to eat more of them! Guavas can have white, pink, red, or yellow pulp. The skin is generally very thick and must be peeled off. There are many varieties and each has its own unique scent and flavor, but they are equal in nutrition. The seeds are perfectly edible so eat them up with the rest of the flesh.

Guavas are:

- super high in vitamin C, containing the most of any fruit
- high in beta-carotene
- high in the antioxidant lycopene and other antioxidants
- high in copper and manganese
- high in fiber
- low in calories

Buy fresh guava that is blemish free. A ripe fruit will give slightly, like an avocado.

Guava season tends to be in spring and summer only. You can buy canned guava at other times.

Store ripe guavas in the fridge.

Peel then slice or cube the guava; eat by itself, or add to fruit salads.

Make guava juice, serve guava with cheese, try guava ice creams and sorbets, or slice into your favorite green salad.

Herbs

Do you eat enough fresh and dried herbs to get the terrific nutritional benefits they offer? With many fresh herbs available in most supermarkets, it's easy to pack more into your daily diet. Use them in lavish quantities as part of a green salad and you will be doing your body, and your taste buds, a great flavor favor.

Herbs are:

- very high in antioxidants
- packed with vitamins and minerals
- a terrific replacement for salt
- a way to increase the bioavailability of antioxidants in greens

Store fresh herbs with snipped stems in a glass of water; basil and parsley prefer room temperature, cilantro prefers the fridge.

Freeze fresh herbs in a single layer inside plastic bags.

Grow your own herbs. Many are easy to grow and are as happy indoors as outdoors.

Make your own pesto and use it abundantly. Try using herbs other than basil to make pesto, too.

Learn how to make your own tabouli. It isn't hard and it packs a great nutritional punch.

Kiwi

This furry little fruit, which is in fact strictly a large berry, has become a favorite around the world in a relatively short time. Kiwi tends to be especially beloved by young children. This is terrific for the kids as it's so good for them. With its mild flavor and attractive green or gold color, it's easy to eat plenty of kiwi!

Kiwi is:

- super high in vitamin C (a single kiwi provides double the amount an adult needs daily)
- very high in the carotenoid lutein, excellent for eye health
- high in many additional antioxidants, plus vitamins K and E
- high in folate and also potassium and copper
- high in fiber

Buy firm, plump fruit with unblemished skin.

Ripen in a paper bag with a banana if necessary.

Warning! Kiwis decompose fairly quickly once ripe, so keep them in the fridge.

Cut a kiwi in half and simply scoop out the flesh with a spoon, then enjoy.

Try kiwi in smoothies, fruit salads, or mixed with yogurt or ice cream.

Use kiwi as a meat tenderizer: Add it to sauces for fish, meat, or poultry.

Lean Pork

Sorry, you'll have to put down that bacon—and the ham too. The healthiest meats from the pig are the completely unprocessed lean cuts. None of the rest of the porcine meat is top quality enough to be described as a superfood. But the lean cuts certainly can be. Lean pork is as low in fat as skinless chicken breast.

Lean pork is:

- a very good source of protein
- high in zinc, with some iron (but not nearly as much as lean red meats or liver)
- super high in thiamine, also known as vitamin B-1, which is essential to normal brain and body function
- a good source of niacin, vitamins B-6 and B-12, selenium, riboflavin, zinc, and omega-3

Buy the lean and trimmed cuts of pork: chops, tenderloin, shoulder, leg, or loin roast.

Cook over a medium heat. Be wary of overcooking. Lean pork is safe to eat without overcooking—enjoy pork at its succulent best with a hint of pink left in the middle.

Substitute lean pork for lamb, beef, or chicken in your favorite recipes. Remember it's always good to eat a wide variety of different foods.

Lean Red Meat

Lean red meat is a superfood that has stood the test of time. From the days of our distant forebears hunting on the plains of Africa, most human populations have been meat eaters. Your body needs protein, and lean red meat can provide it efficiently while adding other vital, health-giving nutrients. Lean red meat includes beef, lamb, goat, and game meats like venison and elk. Don't forget that the body cannot store protein in the way it can fat and carbohydrates, so it needs a good regular supply.

Lean red meat is:
- very high in iron and zinc
- high in vitamin B-12, essential for optimum brain function
- filling and takes a long time to digest, so it's terrific for those wishing to lose weight
- a good source of vitamin A in a form that is excellent for use by the body

Buy organic if you can afford it.

Look for pasture-fed meats. They contain more omega-3 fatty acids.

Before cooking, trim off any visible fat.

Eat meat cooked in many different ways: pan-fried, stewed, grilled. You can even eat meat raw in dishes like steak tartare.

Ideally adults should eat 100 g of lean red meat up to four times a week.

Liver

Now don't make that face. Learn to love liver and you'll never have to worry about being anemic. And you'll be guaranteeing your body a great supply of many other essential nutrients, too. Hunter-gatherers across the globe have prized the liver of their prey for millennia—with very good reason. The standout nutrient in liver is of course iron, with pork liver providing the highest amount. Remember this is heme iron, meaning it's from an animal source, and it is much more easily absorbed than iron from plant sources.

Liver is:

- super high in iron
- super high in A and B vitamins, especially B-12
- very high in folate, zinc, and selenium
- one of the rare natural sources of vitamin D

Cook liver quickly in thin slices, pan-fry, grill, braise, or stew.

Feed it to the family in small portions. Add a few spoonfuls of finely diced liver to pasta sauce, stews, and other meals containing minced or ground beef.

Idea! If you can't bring yourself to cook liver, then make a habit of finding a cafe or restaurant that serves it and enjoy it there. Italian cuisine especially offers several tasty ways of presenting liver.

Mango

Renowned for its sweet perfume and unique flavor, the mango is known as the "king of fruits" for many good reasons. Mangoes are nutrient rich and unlike some other foods are very easy to eat in large quantities. Ask any child! Mangoes are also tremendously versatile; you can use them in so many salads, desserts, and drinks, as well as in their raw, and very delicious, form.

Mango is:

- very high in beta-carotene, the precursor to vitamin A—a whole mango can provide more than three times the recommended daily amount (RDA) of vitamin A
- high in vitamins C and B-6
- high in prebiotic fiber, which is excellent for the gut
- high in polyphenolic antioxidants, known to be protective against some cancers
- a high source of potassium
- a source of copper

Buy mangoes in season; they taste so much better when super fresh.

Use your nose to check if a mango is ripe. It has a distinctive tropical, fruity scent, is firm but not hard, and has an unblemished skin.

Store at room temperature until fully ripe and then in the fridge, but never in a plastic bag.

Babies tend to love mango, making it great to use as a first food.

Milk

Go on, indulge in a glass of milk. It's such an easy way to boost your intake of a few key nutrients. Make the milk low fat and you'll be doing even better. Calcium is the mineral we all associate with milk, and we know how important it is for bones and teeth. But calcium also plays an important role in the workings of nerves and muscles and in making sure blood can clot efficiently. Three servings of dairy foods per day can provide most of the calcium you need, and in its most bioavailable form. There are plenty of other vital nutrients in milk, too, and these are very important for good brain functioning and immune support.

Milk is:

- very high in vitamins D and B-12
- very high in calcium
- high in protein
- high in the B vitamin riboflavin, essential for growth and for healthy eyes and skin
- high in phosphorus, potassium, magnesium, and selenium

Start the day with a smoothie made of low-fat milk and fresh fruit.

Use in baking.

Evaporated milk is delicious in creamy sauces or poured over fresh or canned fruit for a quick dessert.

Add milk to your evening meals in white sauces and frittatas.

Mushrooms

Regarded as a health food for millennia by the Chinese, the nutritional qualities of the many varieties of mushroom and their rich flavor are now far more fully appreciated in the West. Neither a plant nor an animal, mushrooms form a separate food group, the fungi, and have unique properties. The most common forms you will find are white button mushrooms, large white field mushrooms, brown mushrooms, and portobello mushrooms. Just 100 mg a day of mushrooms has been shown to reduce the risk of breast and prostate cancer.

Mushrooms are:
- very low in calories
- known to stimulate the immune system
- a good source of selenium, potassium, riboflavin, niacin, and vitamin D
- a source of bulk in the diet and help you feel full

Buy mushrooms fresh, or pick wild ones if you are *sure* you know which ones are edible.

Store in the fridge, in the cling-wrapped packaging they came in or in a brown paper bag.

Roast button mushrooms whole in a hot oven; slice and stir-fry; add to salads, stews, and casseroles; or make mushroom soups.

Eat mushrooms for breakfast, to start your day the nutrition-packed way.

Enjoy the texture of mushrooms as much as the flavor.

Oats

The Scots have known it for centuries: Oats really are the best of the best when it comes to complex carbohydrates. Oats are a slow-burn food, keeping you full for a long time and filling you up with a great range of nutrients.

Oats are:

- very high in a soluble fiber called beta-glucan, which is why they lower blood cholesterol
- high in E and B vitamins, potassium, calcium, iron, zinc, and selenium
- a very-low-GI carbohydrate
- high in protein compared to other cereals
- a source of healthy unsaturated fats
- gluten free, or almost gluten free—this debate is unresolved

Store oats in an airtight container.

Buy rolled oats, they are far superior to instant oats.

Eat oats as hot cereal and as oat cakes.

Try oatmeal with salt and a little butter, or with brown sugar and raspberries, or pear and cinnamon.

Make your own superfoods muesli with oats, nuts, and a small amount of dried fruits. Add ground flaxseed and spices, and reap the nutritional benefits.

Bake biscuits and pancakes with oats, and use oats to make crumble toppings for fruit.

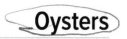

Oysters

Don't faint, just take a deep breath and get your head around the idea of increasing your oyster intake. Your body will thank you for it. This marvelous mollusk is the richest source of zinc of any food on the planet. Oysters are not just high in zinc, they are also high on the list of super-foods. But zinc is not the only nutrient abundant in this brilliant bivalve.

Oysters are:

- the best known source of the mineral zinc. One oyster has 10 mg of zinc, while a dozen will give you about ten times your daily needs
- high in iron, magnesium, phosphorus, selenium, iodine, and copper
- an excellent source of vitamins D and B-12
- low in calories and fat

Buy oysters as fresh as possible.

Store in the fridge but *not* in water.

Serve on the half shell on a bed of ice with lemon on the side.

Eat raw. Oh, go on, slurp them down. A bit of lemon, salt, and pepper is all you need.

Bake, smoke, boil, fry, roast, stew, steam, or broil them, too.

Try canned smoked oysters for a quick zinc hit.

Drink oysters as a cocktail with a bloody mary or tequila. Go on!

Do eat them to improve your love life. Oysters reportedly contain amino acids and high levels of zinc, both of which trigger increased levels of the sex hormone testosterone.

Passionfruit

Get some passion back into the kitchen with this lip-smackingly tasty fruit. The passionfruit is a nutrient-dense fruit that is used far too sparingly. Most often seen in its purple form, passionfruit can also be yellow, gold, red, or the larger red Panama variety. They are all nutritionally equal.

Passionfruit is:
- super high in soluble fiber, higher than any other fruit
- high in beta-carotene, the precursor to vitamin A
- high in vitamin C
- a good source of B vitamins and iron

Buy fruit that feels heavy for its size, with unwrinkled skin.

Store at room temperature for two weeks or in the fridge for four weeks—store in a plastic bag to prevent the fruit from drying out.

Freeze the pulp in ice cube trays or small containers.

Don't just use passionfruit as a decoration for desserts or fruit salads; make it the main fruit in your dish.

Do eat the fruit just as it is. Simply cut the passionfruit in half and eat the pulp and seeds with a spoon. Kids love it like this!

Blend into smoothies for breakfast, mix with yogurt and cream for dessert, make passionfruit curd and spread it liberally onto toast, or stir it into plain yogurt.

Grow your own passionfruit vine, it's surprisingly easy.

Peas

Peas bestride two food groups, like the nutritional colossus they are. They are both vegetables and legumes. They have the higher protein content of beans and similar amounts of fiber, but they are more digestible. Sugar snap and snow peas include the pods of the peas, and are definitely vegetables.

Peas are:

- high in vitamins C and K and the B vitamins
- high in manganese, magnesium, iron, zinc, and potassium
- high in soluble and insoluble fiber, excellent for the gut
- high in cancer-fighting antioxidants, which are also excellent for eye health

Buy peas frozen, keep it simple! Frozen peas tend to be much cheaper than fresh—peas are frozen within a couple of hours of being picked so all the nutrients get frozen in fast.

Cook frozen peas very quickly, it only takes three minutes.

Lightly steam sugar snap and snow peas, or eat them raw; they are delicious this way, especially in salads.

Peas are so versatile, you can eat them as a simple vegetable or as the basis for soups and stews—add them to casseroles, salads, and stir-fries.

Experiment with pea guacamole, mash peas with potatoes, or add to pasta sauces.

Peppers

Peppers pack a punch, and not just for the tastebuds. Both bell peppers and the smaller, more-fiery chili peppers are full of antioxidants and a range of vitamins and minerals. Chilies are in fact the more nutritious, but it can be hard to eat a large amount of them! Do try to up your intake though; get used to the burn and you'll set your metabolism on fire. Red, yellow, orange, and purple bell peppers are much easier to eat in large quantities and yield plenty of great nutrients.

Peppers are:
- high in beta-carotene
- high in fiber
- high in vitamins C and K, plus the B vitamins
- high in potassium, manganese, and magnesium
- high in antioxidants
- a great way to boost the metabolism (especially chilies)

Buy peppers with smooth, taut skins and even color.

Store in the fridge, or chop up and freeze for longer-term storage.

Choose red peppers rather than green, as they have more nutritional oomph.

Make pepper soups, ratatouille, and stews, or caramelize with onions.

Be generous when you add peppers to stir-fries, chili con carne, soups, and stews.

Add chili to desserts! Try chili-chocolate brownies, choco-chili ice cream, and chili-lime mango.

Pomegranates

The rich, ruby-red color of these succulent fruits signals that they are incredibly good for us. Like all deeply colored fruits and vegetables, pomegranates are packed full of health-promoting and cancer-fighting antioxidants. Within its leathery skin, the pomegranate holds hundreds of juicy red "arils," each with a small pip inside. The distinctive taste of the pomegranate lends itself to many dishes as well as to simply being eaten plain. As they are generally only available in autumn, gorge yourselves on pomegranate when you can!

Pomegranates are:

- super high in the protective antioxidants known as polyphenols
- high in vitamin C and potassium
- high in fiber
- low in calories

Buy firm pomegranates that feel heavy and whose skin is taut.

Store at room temperature for a few days. They'll keep for two to three months when refrigerated in a plastic bag.

Better to buy and eat the whole fruit than to simply drink bottled pomegranate juice.

Savory dishes get a real boost from adding pomegranate; use it in a stuffing for chicken or in a sauce or glaze for red meats.

Bake pomegranates into muffins and cakes, or try pomegranate compote.

Make your own pomegranate juice by blending the arils and straining the juice.

Raspberries

Sink your teeth into some ruby-red raspberries and you'll enjoy not just the flavors but also the terrific health benefits of this sweet, luscious fruit.

Raspberries are:

- super high in fiber (100 g of raspberries has just over 6 g of fiber compared to a slice of whole-grain bread, which has only 2.5 g)
- high in many antioxidants, including several that help fight inflammation, cancer, and aging
- very rich in the anthocyanins
- high in vitamins A, C, E, and K, plus the B vitamins
- a good source of potassium, manganese, copper, iron, and magnesium
- very low in calories

Buy fresh and in season, or pick your own if there's a farm near you.

Choose deep red, shiny fruit that look firm and plump.

Store in the fridge, but not for long as raspberries spoil quickly.

Buy frozen all year round. Frozen berries are generally much cheaper than fresh but have all the same nutrients intact.

Enjoy a couple of handfuls for breakfast with cereal or in smoothies; try in vegetable salads, too.

Pack homemade ice cream with raspberries, or mix lots of frozen raspberries with slightly thawed store-bought ice cream.

Quinoa

Like chia, quinoa is a seed that is treated as more of a grain. Both are from South America and have been cultivated there for many thousands of years. Quinoa was known as the "mother of all grains." Quinoa comes in grey, black, and white varieties, with white being the most common. It looks and behaves a bit like couscous but packs more of a nutritional punch. A gluten-free food, quinoa is increasingly recognized as a valuable food because of its overall nutritional richness. Perhaps that's not a surprise when you consider it comes from the same family as spinach.

Quinoa is:

- high in protein, including lysine, an essential amino acid unusual in plant foods—in fact, quinoa contains complete protein, unlike most grains
- a low-GI food
- high in iron, B vitamins, and potassium
- high in fiber
- mineral dense, especially in manganese, phosphorus, and magnesium
- a good source of antioxidants

Buy it in bulk. Go on, it's good for you.

Store in airtight containers; keeps longer in the fridge.

Cook by boiling for approximately 15 minutes and then fluff with a fork—use stock instead of water for extra taste.

Great for breakfast and as an alternative to potatoes, rice, or pasta.

Bake into cakes and cookies.

Salmon and Other Oily Fish

Known for millennia as a "brain food," salmon and other oily fish really are nutritional powerhouses. Science has finally caught up with traditional wisdom to explain why the oils found in salmon can keep the brain and body healthy and working at their best. Eat these fish twice weekly; they are quick and easy to cook and taste delicious. In most Western countries the majority of the population do not eat nearly as much fish as is advisable. So grab your shopping basket, or a fishing line, and get some salmon today!

Salmon and other oily fish are:

- some of the richest sources of omega-3 fats
- protein packed
- low in saturated fats
- rich in zinc
- high in iodine; potassium; vitamins A, B, and D; copper; iron; and selenium
- a source of calcium

Buy very fresh, or frozen (for convenience). Most salmon is farmed, but watch for wild salmon, too.

Store in the fridge or freezer, but eat quickly.

Eat at least twice a week. Steam, BBQ, pan-fry, use in pies or frittatas, with pasta, in stir-fries, and in salads—eat hot or cold.

Did you know? Salmon can jump up to six feet into the air when swimming upriver.

Seafood: Mollusks and Crustaceans

Three cheers for the mighty mollusks and the cool crustaceans! Seafood is really good for us, and preparing it is simple. Mussels, shrimp, crawfish, clams, scallops, octopus, squid, lobster, crab, and abalone are all superfoods because of their superhigh levels of nutrition. These animals are more nutritious than red meat: They have more protein, most have less fat, and they have lots more minerals. Some types have more protein and less fat than even skinless chicken breast. Note that squid, fish roe, shrimp, and prawns can be high in cholesterol.

Shellfish are:

- super high in protein, and low in fat overall with good amounts of omega-3 fatty acids
- very rich in iron and zinc—mussels and octopus have twice as much iron as beef!
- rich in magnesium, manganese, phosphorous, selenium, calcium, and B vitamins
- low in calories

Buy from a fishmonger with a high turnover, or buy frozen.

Start your seafood-cooking adventure with garlic prawns, simple and delicious, then take it from there.

Try seafood chowder, then crab cakes, mussels in white wine, bouillabaisse, and on and yummily on!

Eat a wide variety of seafood to reap all the benefits of their various nutrients.

Seaweed

Many types of seaweed can be eaten, and although they can look very different, all seaweeds belong to the algae family. Coastal people from all over the world have always eaten seaweed, and for very good reason. The common edible types are *nori,* the sheets wrapped around sushi; *arame,* sold in stringlike strips; *dulse,* a strong-flavored seaweed; *hijiki,* a mild, almost sweet seaweed; *kombu,* a type of kelp; and *wakame,* a tender, deep green seaweed. Much research is looking at the benefits of seaweeds for those needing to lose weight. It looks promising! Go on, try a little seaweed, and if you like it, eat a lot.

Seaweed is:

- high in iodine, especially kombu
- high in B vitamins, plus vitamins C and E, and also folate
- high in magnesium, calcium, and boron
- a useful source of iron and phosphorus
- high in antioxidants

Find seaweed in Asian stores and in health-food shops, where it is usually sold dried.

Add seaweeds to soups, stir-fries, and salads, and use them in and around homemade sushi.

Spices

Researchers are toiling away in laboratories all over the world, proving the health benefits of spices. Spices are chock full of powerful antioxidants and have many health-giving properties, and scientists are finally realizing what people throughout the world have believed for millennia. Many spices are also rich in minerals and vitamins, but since most of us eat only small amounts of spices, can they make a difference? The answer is yes, so it's a great idea to up your spice intake in general.

Spices offer the following benefits, and more:

- cinnamon, only ½ teaspoon a day, can help keep blood sugar low
- ginger can reduce nausea, joint inflammation, and pain
- turmeric reduces inflammation and can inhibit cancer growth
- garlic kills off viruses and bacteria

Cook more spicy dishes; give your taste buds a treat.

Add some turmeric and other spices to the water when you cook rice.

Drink more chai tea. And you don't need to add sugar, as the spices "sweeten" the drink.

Add more fresh ginger, garlic, and pepper to your stir-fries.

Bake more cakes, biscuits, and puddings with cinnamon, cardamom, nutmeg, and ginger.

Spinach

Take a bow you leafy green queen of the superfoods. Spinach is so good for us: Can't you just tell from the bright green color of its leaves? Spinach may be green and leafy and look a bit weedy and insubstantial, but it packs a Popeye-powerful punch when it comes to nutrition.

Spinach is:

- high in iron, magnesium, calcium, manganese, zinc, and potassium
- high in vitamins A, C, B-6, K, and E
- full of fiber
- an antioxidant hit, with lutein and beta-carotene and others that promote eye health
- very low in calories, so enjoy spinach by the truckload

Buy fresh or frozen, both are equally nutritious.

Grow your own, as spinach is easy to grow even in cool climates.

Store in the fridge in a plastic bag or sealed container. If you need to wash spinach, do so just before cooking.

Eat in copious quantities in salads with a healthy fat, which helps the body absorb all the nutrients.

Add a cup of baby spinach to a smoothie.

Cook in frittatas, omelettes, and stir-fries.

Add to soups, pasta sauce, lasagne, stews, and casseroles.

Sweet Potato

Like most vegetables, the more colorful the better when it comes to this terrific tuber. So choose deep-orange sweet potatoes and reap the health-giving benefits. Start the kids on sweet potatoes when they're young and steer them away from white potato chips and fries.

Sweet potato is:
- high in fiber
- high in vitamins A, C, and B-6
- high in potassium and manganese
- a lower-GI food than white potatoes, and the GI is lowest when boiled rather than baked

Store in a cool, dark, and well-ventilated place.

Swap sweet potatoes for your regular white potatoes. Immediately!

Roast them whole or cut into cubes and toss with salt, pepper, olive oil, and herbs or cinnamon.

Bake them in foil and top with cottage cheese. Mash them with a little butter, milk, and nutmeg.

Eat the skin of the sweet potato; it has great nutrients and fiber and is perfectly edible.

Excellent in curries and in soups. Try a recipe using sweet potato in a cake, too!

Kids tend to love sweet potato. Make sweet potato chips by slicing thin and brushing with olive oil; bake for ten minutes, turn over, and bake for another ten.

Tea: Black, Green, and White

Brew a cup of tea, and you have in your hands a warm cup of steaming antioxidants. (But hold the sugar, please.) The benefits of a good cup of tea are now widely recognized, and in tea's case it's all about quantity as well as quality. Tea may have fewer antioxidants than some other foods (for example, cloves contain more polyphenols), but it's a lot more pleasant to drink a few cups of tea than to eat 100 grams of cloves. All types of tea come from the same plant. For black tea the leaves are crushed and fermented, for green they are dried then steamed, for white they are simply steamed.

Tea is:

- very rich in polyphenols, which seek and destroy free radicals
- apparently a cancer fighter
- preventive against heart disease, stroke, and bad cholesterol
- low in calories yet boosts the metabolism to burn energy faster
- a source of both caffeine and theanine, which stimulate the brain

All caffeinated tea is good tea; green and black tea appear equally beneficial. Decaf tea is only beneficial if a natural water process is used, as it retains the tea's antioxidants.

Stick to four or five cups of tea a day and you will not have to worry about overconsuming caffeine.

Tomatoes

There's nothing humble about the tomato. This excellent fruit, yes fruit, is chock full of antioxidants. It's a cancer killer, especially when cooked, and as a paste it is super high in lycopene, a terrific antioxidant. The orange and yellow tomatoes are as good for you as the rich, deep red ones; they contain a different but equally powerful type of lycopene. Now available in a vast variety of shapes and sizes, tomatoes should be a firm fixture in your daily diet.

Tomatoes are:
- the richest source of lycopene on the planet
- high in fiber
- high in vitamins C, K, E, and B-6
- rich in essential minerals
- famed as a terrific food for heart health
- very low in calories

Buy as fresh as possible and in any varieties you like.

Store at room temperature; put them in the fruit bowl.

Don't forget canned, dried, and paste.

Grow easily in sunny spots in spring and summer.

Kids tend to love tomatoes, especially the small cherry and grape varieties. Make them a tomato skewer with beets and cucumber, or give them whole to eat like apples.

Cook in almost every dish you care to mention, and don't forget to simply roast or fry them. They are ideal as a breakfast treat.

Walnuts

The whole nut looks like the human skull, and when you crack it open the nut itself looks like a brain! They don't look like the human brain for nothing: Walnuts are a terrific brain food. Walnuts are the nuts with the most long-chain polyunsaturated fats. And you only need a small serving each day to reap the benefits.

Walnuts are:

- helpful in lowering bad cholesterol and raising good cholesterol
- high in omega-3 fatty acids (a 30 g serving gives you 90 percent of the recommended daily intake)
- high in antioxidants, especially polyphenolic compounds—scientists say they contain twice as many antioxidants as other nuts
- high in vitamins B and D, and folic acid
- high in manganese, copper, potassium, calcium, iron, magnesium, zinc, and selenium
- a good source of fiber and protein

Buy as fresh as possible, from shops with a high turnover, or in sealed packs from the supermarket.

Eat just 28 g a day for a nutrient boost.

Store in the fridge, and chop them only as needed.

Use in salads, add small amounts to fruit smoothies, and bake into bread, brownies, and cakes.

Try walnut sauces for chicken, walnut pesto, walnut hummus, and candied walnuts.

Tastiest when toasted in a hot oven for just a few minutes.

Whitefish

Although salmon and the other oily fish usually hog the healthy-eating limelight, please do not underestimate the nonoily species of whitefish. Whitefish like snapper, Asian seabass, halibut, cod, mahi mahi, haddock, sole, and flounder are terrific sources of protein, are very low in saturated fats, and are rich in vitamins and minerals. Make the whitefish species a weekly feature on your menu plan, and your body and brain will thank you for it.

Whitefish are:

- very high in protein
- high in niacin, vitamins B-6 and B-12, phosphorus, and selenium
- low in fat

Choose fresh fish with bright red gills; bright, clear eyes; clean, shiny skin; and a pleasant, briny smell.

Or buy frozen—flash frozen and vacuum sealed is by the far the best.

Store in the fridge, on top of crushed ice if possible.

Wrap fish in wet newspaper or baking paper and bake in the oven.

Stew it. Whitefish make excellent fish stews that are especially tasty if you add some delicious shellfish.

Fish pies topped with pastry or mashed potato are often popular with kids.

Yogurt

I'm not talking about the sugary confection that poses as yogurt on many supermarket shelves. The health-giving yogurt that can protect your body from all sorts of nasties is the most natural yogurt you can get, the plain and deliciously creamy, delectable sort. And go full fat for extra taste and yumminess; it won't kill you. It's the good bacteria that your body will benefit from. Good, natural yogurt is teeming with minimicrobes, or probiotics, that can really enhance your gut flora.

Yogurt is:
- high in protective microbes
- high in calcium, protein, and B vitamins
- very easily digested by the body (your body absorbs more nutrients from yogurt than from an equivalent amount of milk)
- yogurts and other low-fat milk products are now proven to play a useful part in weight loss

Buy the best natural yogurt, you deserve it.

Make your own yogurt. It is easy to do at home and you need never run out.

Eat yogurt daily to keep topping up the good bacteria in your digestive tract.

Add your own fruit, jam, nuts, seeds, honey, maple syrup, or even a dash of sugar.

Make healthy dips using yogurt as a base.

Cook with yogurt. Add it to stews and soups, and bake it into cakes and cookies.

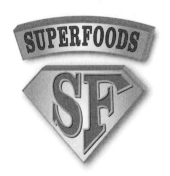

THE BEST
OF THE REST

Breads

Choose anything except plain white bread—anything!! Seriously, there are so many other great-tasting options, why bother with plain white?

Try instead:

- sourdough bread, even white sourdough bread. It's a much-lower GI food than plain white bread
- rye and whole-grain sourdough; they are much more nutritious
- whole-grain bread; get all the nutrition from a grain of wheat
- dark rye bread, often known as pumpernickel, which is a low-GI food and comes in handy small servings
- whole-grain pita breads and flat breads

Drinks

Water is a popular drink that has stood the test of time. It's refreshing and calorie free!

Herbal teas.

Smoothies made from low-fat milk, yogurt, and superfood fruits. Hold the ice cream!

Vegetable juices. Freshly juiced is best; add some ginger for extra zing.

Cocoa made with real cocoa powder and low-fat milk.

Skim milk.

Mixed fruit and vegetable juices. Get the kids used to these first, and then switch to vegetable only.

Whole fruit juices. Try blending whole fruit with ice and water in a powerful blender.

Pure fruit juices, in moderation.

Red wine—a glass a day will do the trick.

Fruits

There are so many fruits in the Top 50 Superfoods, and they are the ones that stand tallest nutritionally. But all fruits are beneficial. Feel free to eat widely and eat well when it comes to fruits.

Those that are better for you include:

- apples
- apricots
- bananas
- cantaloupe
- cherries
- cranberries
- grapes
- honeydew melon
- lychees
- papaya
- peaches
- pears
- persimmons
- pineapples
- plums
- watermelon

Grains and Cereals

Eat:
- brown rice
- bulgur/cracked wheat
- corn flakes
- corn tortillas
- couscous
- enriched white bread
- multigrain bread
- popcorn—plain
- wheat cereal
- whole-wheat crackers
- whole-wheat cereal
- whole-wheat noodles

Avoid:
- processed white bread
- white rice

Nuts

All nuts are pretty good for us because they're a source of good fats and protein. Nuts also have fiber and will keep you feeling fuller longer, plus they appear to boost serotonin levels. But exercise restraint, a handful a day is as many as you need.

Brazil nuts
- are super high in selenium; a single nut can give you your ideal daily dose

Cashews
- are high in magnesium, having even more than almonds. Also high in iron and zinc

Hazelnuts
- are a good source of iron and a group of antioxidants named proanthocyanidins; highest in fiber

Peanuts
- are high in folate (they are strictly a legume but can be classified as a nut, nutritionally speaking)

Pine nuts
- are a source of omega-6 fats and are high in zinc, iron, folate, and fiber

Pistachios
- are an excellent source of potassium; high in cholesterol-lowering plant sterols

Protein Sources

There are so many good sources of protein that choosing can be difficult. Just steer clear of meats with a high fat content.

Nuts—*see* Nuts (opposite)

Cheese—the lower-fat varieties like cottage cheese and ricotta are best. Eat the higher-fat cheeses in moderation

Fish—grilled, broiled, smoked, but not deep fried. Tuna is a good source of protein, canned or fresh

Pork—all lean cuts

Seafood—prawns, shrimp, crab

Seeds—pumpkin or sunflower

Tofu or tempeh

Turkey—all lean cuts

Vegetables

All vegetables are good for you. The main message here is to eat vegetables abundantly, in vast quantities, as many as you can manage. Your waistline will thank you. So will your intestines. The fiber in veggies is good for the gut and for the beneficial gut microbes that live there.

- Think vibrant colors; make a rainbow on your plate.
- Eat vegetables raw as well as cooked, as both ways afford benefits.

Boost Your Nutrient Intake

If you need *B vitamins,* sprinkle *wheatgerm* over your breakfast cereal or add it to your smoothies or baking, or eat some *beef liver.*

If you need *vitamin C,* eat *guavas* or *kiwis.*

If you need *zinc,* eat fresh or canned, smoked *oysters.*

If you need *iron,* eat *liver, beans (especially soy), tofu, mussels, whole grains, oysters,* or *red meat* and *all dark green, leafy vegetables, such as spinach.*

If you need *fiber,* eat *kiwi fruit, chia, flaxseeds,* and *raspberries.*

If you need *vitamin B-12,* eat *oysters, clams, mussels, liver, fish, meat,* and *eggs.*

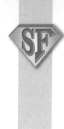

Websites

General Superfoods Website

Nutrient Rich Foods Coalition

www.nutrientrichfoods.org

Check out the website of the Nutrient Rich Foods Coalition, which is a U.S.-based partnership of scientists, health professionals, communication experts, and agricultural organizations. It aims to inform and inspire people to improve their diets by eating more nutrient-dense foods, and, by association, fewer nutritionally poor foods. Their website contains information and downloadable items for both health professionals and consumers.

You will find:
- a shopping list of nutrient-rich foods
- a guide to nutrition labels
- information on portions
- advice on fitting in "fun" foods
- recipes
- meal plans

Other Recommended Nutrition Websites

Foodwatch

www.foodwatch.com.au

Australian accredited nutritionist and dietician Catherine Saxelby provides a wealth of information on eating well. Her well-balanced, expert approach is very reliable, and her recipes are delicious. She is the author of several influential books.

Dr. Joanna

www.drjoanna.com.au

Dr. Joanna McMillan is an Australian nutritionist and dietician whose website is packed with ideas and advice on healthy eating. There are terrific healthy and delicious recipes and information about her books.

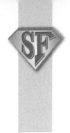

Sources of Great Superfood Recipes

If you are looking for some fantastic recipes using whole superfoods, then take a look at the websites of the organizations that promote the foods.

Here are some to get you started. Do an online search for any of the superfoods.

California Almonds
www.almondboard.com

California Asparagus Commission
www.calasparagus.com
Did you know that 70 percent of the asparagus cultivated in the United States is grown in California?

American Egg Board
www.aeb.org

California Walnuts Commission
www.walnuts.org

Oregon Blueberry Commission
www.oregonblueberry.com

Author Bio

Seana Smith was born and brought up in Scotland. She now lives in Sydney, Australia, with her hungry husband and four ravenous and very active children.

Seana is the author or coauthor of three previous books, all published in Australia by Jane Curry Publishing:

- *Sydney for Under Fives*
- *The Australian Autism Handbook* (1st edition)
- *Beyond the Baby Blues*

Seana blogs at: Sydney, Kids, Food + Travel (www.seana smith.com). Blog topics include:

- the best of Sydney for kids
- family-friendly recipes
- family travel
- life balance and mental health

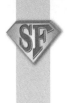

Index